WALK IT OUT

(A Walking For Weight Loss Guide for Nigerians)

'Denike Owolabi

Walk It Out

Ordering Details

To place orders or for details of discounts for bulk purchases by organizations or groups either for support, gift, training packages, fundraising, or any other educational purposes, send an email to denikeowolabi65@gmail.com.

Table of Contents

Dedication

This book is dedicated to all individuals on their weight loss journey, embracing the challenge and taking charge of their health, regardless of their size. You are not alone in this pursuit, and together, we can achieve our goals and create positive changes in our lives.

Acknowledgement

I extend my deepest appreciation to my family for their unwavering support as I put this ebook together. To my husband, your encouragement on my weight loss journey, your love, and your active participation in exercise and walks have been my pillars of strength. I thank my daughter, Timi, for her creative brainstorming sessions on the book title and valuable contributions throughout the writing process.

A special acknowledgment to my dedicated proofreader and editor, Pst (Mrs) Modupe Oyedele. Your meticulous attention to detail ensured the precision and clarity of every word, and your insightful suggestions significantly enhanced the quality of this work. Thank you for your exceptional contributions.

Foreword

Welcome to the beginning of an extraordinary journey towards a healthier, more vibrant you! This book is more than just a guide on walking for weight loss; it's a companion cheering you on every step of the way.

In these pages, you'll find practical advice wrapped in understanding and empathy. It's not just about shedding pounds; it's about transforming your entire self. The author shares not only wisdom but a personal story of struggles, victories, and a shift in self-perception.

Let these words be the motivation to tie those shoelaces, step outside, and embark on a journey that goes beyond the physical act of walking. It's a quest for a healthier lifestyle, a journey to self-love, and a celebration of the incredible person that is you.

The journey awaits, and within these pages,

you have a trusted companion for every single
step.

Pst Omotola OwolabiPresiding Pastor
Restoration-Word Of Harvest Worldwide

Disclaimer

The information provided in this book is based on personal experiences, research, and general knowledge. Before making any significant changes to your diet or lifestyle, it is advisable to consult with a qualified healthcare professional or nutritionist. The author and publisher are not responsible for any consequences resulting from the implementation of the advice and suggestions in this book.

Introduction

My Journey Towards Weight Loss

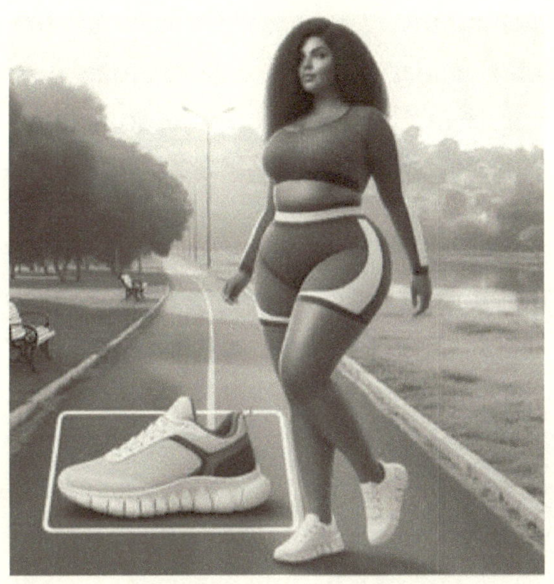

Created with Microsoft Bing AI Image Creator

From the moment I became aware of myself as a girl, I also became conscious of the weight that seemed so cling to me like an uninvited companion. It wasn't something I could ignore or brush aside even if I had wanted to. Where I come from, there is always a name to refer to plus size individuals, both young and old; it was ever-present, demanding my attention and somewhat affecting my self-esteem.

No one knew this, but the burden of watching my weight was a heavy one to bear at such a tender age. One I bore alone, constantly being reminded that there was something about me that needed to be fixed.

As I grew older, I realised that my weight was not just a physical issue but an emotional one too. It became a constant source of insecurity and self-doubt. I couldn't help but compare myself to others, wondering why it was so effortless for them to maintain a slimmer figure while I struggled with every bite I took.

Watching my weight soon turned into an obsession. Every meal became a battleground of conflicting emotions - the desire to enjoy food clashing with the guilt of potential weight gain. I couldn't escape the ever-present fear of judgment, imagining that others were silently scrutinizing my body.

The pursuit of weight loss became a rollercoaster of hope and disappointment. I'd celebrate small victories, only to stumble and find myself back where I started. It felt like an uphill battle I couldn't conquer.

I vividly recall expressing my frustrations to a close family friend, but little did I know that their response would leave a lasting impact on me. They pointed out the weight of my close relatives, all of whom were plus-size, and made me realise that my own weight was lower because of my consciousness and efforts. In that moment, I felt a sense of accomplishment, I was winning the battle against high body weight.

At times, I resorted to extreme measures, hoping for a quick fix. Crash diets and intense exercise regimens left me feeling exhausted and defeated. I had to come to terms with the fact that there was no magic solution, no overnight transformation.

As I matured, I learned that the journey to a healthier self was not just about the number on the scale; it was about finding balance and acceptance. I began to focus on nourishing my body with wholesome foods, learning to listen to its needs.

Gradually, I shifted my perspective from viewing my weight as a measure of my worth to embracing the unique person I was - regardless of my size. I discovered that my weight didn't define me, and it certainly shouldn't limit me to be whatever I want to be.

The journey to watch my weight is still a part of my life, but it no longer consumes me. I've come to understand that it's okay to have moments of vulnerability and imperfection. What matters is my commitment to taking care of myself and nurturing my well-being.

I have found strength in my experiences. I know that I am not alone in this battle and that manyothers face similar challenges. My hope is that my story will reach those who, like me, have struggled with their weight since they were young, and that they will find solace in knowing that they are not alone.

I am no longer that young girl who felt burdened by her weight. Today, I stand as a woman who has learned to love herself, flaws and all. One who has learned to ignore family, friends and acquaintances whose first words to you always is "you have gained weight or you are gaining weight", not caring to know your story and how depressing such words can be. Of course, there are times such remarks serve as a wake-up call to be mindful of one's health, they can also be hurtful and lacking in sensitivity and love.

Interestingly, I must admit that, I too, have occasionally been guilty of pointing out others' weight. I realise now how my words might have been perceived, and I genuinely apologise if I ever came across as insensitive. It's essential for all of us to be more mindful of the impact our words can have on others and to choose our language with kindness and empathy.

I understand that this path is essential for my overall health and vitality. With each step forward, I grow stronger and more committed to the pursuit of a healthier and happier me. I am determined to continue this journey, not just for the physical transformation, but for the positive impact it has on my well-being and quality of life.

Learning to love oneself, regardless of body size, is a continuous journey of self-acceptance and growth. Let us strive to uplift and support each other, focusing on the beauty within us beyond physical appearances. Together, we can create a more compassionate and understanding environment where everyone feels valued and loved, just as they are.

Walk It Out!

Walking Works For Me

In the pursuit of managing my weight, I embarked on a journey that took me down many paths - some rocky, some smooth. I had tried various diets, exercise regimens, and weight loss programs, but none seemed to offer a lasting solution. Frustration and disappointment were myconstant companions.

It wasn't until one unassuming day that I stumbled upon a simple yet transformative solution - walking. As I laced up my sneakers and stepped outside, I had no inkling of the profound impact this straightforward activity would have on my life.

At first, walking was just a means to get some fresh air and clear my mind. Little did I know that those leisurely strolls would turn into a powerful tool for weight management. As I continued my walks, I began to notice changes in my body and mindset. The pounds didn't magically disappear overnight, but something within me shifted.

I decided to dig deeper into the science behind walking for weight management. To my surprise, I discovered that this seemingly ordinary activity had a plethora of benefits. Walking not only burned calories but also revved up my metabolism and helped regulate my appetite. It was like unlocking a hidden potential within my body that had been waiting to be unleashed.

Armed with this newfound knowledge, I set

out to make the most of my walking routine. Gradually, I increased the intensity and duration of my walks, challenging myself to push beyond my comfort zone.

Walking became more than just an exercise; it became a journey of self-discovery and empowerment. I discovered I don't even have to leave the comfort of my home to walk as I found joy in exploring new walking workouts on YouTube. Each step is an affirmation of my commitment to a healthier and happier life.

One of the most transformative elements of my walking journey has been the support network I established. I sort for like-minded individuals who shared similar goals, and I initiated "Walk To Fitness" on social media. Through this group, I post videos of walking workouts to motivate and inspire members to walk daily. The sense of community that has blossomed around this initiative has uplifted me in ways I never expected.

Being part of such a supportive and encouraging group has been a driving force in my walking success and has made the journey even more enjoyable and fulfilling.

Not So Smooth

The path of weight management wasn't always smooth. I encountered plateaus and setbacks, but I learned to embrace them as part of the journey. With persistence and determination, I navigated through these challenges, knowing that each step brought me closer to my goals.

I have resolved to make walking a lifelong habit, an integral part of my daily routine. It is no longer a means to an end but a journey I will be committed to for the rest of my life. It isn't about a destination; it is about embracing the process and the person I am becoming along the way.

As I reflect on my walking journey, I am grateful for the simplicity and power it brought into my life. I had unlocked a solution that had always been within reach. Walking isn't a quick fix or a trendy fad; it is a timeless activity that has the potential to transform lives - including mine.

So, to anyone on their own weight management journey, I say this: lace up your sneakers and take that first step. Embrace the simplicity of walking, for within it lies the power to discover a healthier, happier, and more fulfilled version of yourself. The path may not always be easy, but each step is a testament to your strength and commitment. Walk on, and may you find the beauty and transformation that I found on this incredible journey.

Walk It Out!

Benefits Of Walking For Weight Loss

Walking is a timeless and accessible activity that offers a wide range of benefits for weight loss. Whether you're just starting your weight loss journey or looking for a sustainable way to shed those extra pounds, incorporating walking into your routine can be a game-changer. Here are some of the remarkable benefits of walking for weight loss:

1. Burns calories: Walking is a low-impact aerobic exercise that can help you burn calories and contribute to creating a calorie deficit. The more calories you burn, the more likely you are to lose weight, especially when combined with a balanced diet.

2. Boosts metabolism: Regular walking can boost your metabolism, even after you finish your walk. This means that your body continues to burn calories at an increased rate, even during periods of rest, aiding in weight loss.

3. Supports fat loss: Walking primarily taps into your body's fat stores for energy during low-intensity activities. As you engage in longer walks, your body gradually shifts to using fat as its primary fuel source, facilitating fat loss and inch reduction.

4. Preserves lean muscle Mass: Unlike some high-intensity exercises, walking helps preserve lean muscle mass while targeting fat loss. This is essential for

maintaining a healthy metabolism and preventing muscle loss during weight loss efforts.

5. Improves cardiovascular health: Walking is an excellent cardiovascular exercise that strengthens your heart and improves blood circulation. A healthy cardiovascular system is crucial for overall well-being and can support your weight loss journey.

6. Reduces stress and emotional eating: Walking has been shown to reduce stress and anxiety, which are common triggers for emotional eating. By incorporating walking into your daily routine, you may find yourself less prone to turning to food for comfort.

7. Enhances mood and mental clarity: Walking releases endorphins, the "feel-good" hormones, which can improve your mood and boost mental clarity. A positive mindset is essential for staying motivated and committed to your weight loss goals.

8. Sustainable and inclusive: walking is a low-impact exercise that is suitable for people of all fitness levels and ages. It can be easily incorporated into your daily routine without the need for expensive equipment or gym memberships, making it a sustainable weight loss strategy.

9. Supports long-term weight maintenance: Unlike extreme diets or intense workouts, walking isa habit that you can maintain over the long term. Consistency is key to weight loss success, and walking offers a practical and enjoyable way to stay committed to your goals.

10. Promotes overall well-being: Beyond weight loss, walking contributes to your overall well-being. It improves sleep quality, boosts energy levels, and enhances your sense of overall health and vitality.

In conclusion, walking is a simple yet powerful tool for weight loss that offers numerous physical, mental, and emotional benefits. By making walking a regular part of your lifestyle, you can create positive changes in your body and mind, supporting your weight loss journey and achieving lasting results. So, put on your walking shoes, step outside, and experience the transformation that walking can bring to your life.

When you cannot step outside, video resources are available online to help you walk in the comfort of your home. No excuses.

A Guide For Nigerians

Walking is not only a universal exercise but also an incredibly suitable one for Nigerians, given the country's diverse landscape, cultural norms, and lifestyle. Here are several reasons why walking is an excellent and well-suited exercise for Nigerians:

1. Accessible and inclusive: Walking requires no special equipment or facilities, making it accessible to people of all ages and fitness levels. Whether

you live in a bustling city or a rural area, you can engage in walking as a form of exercise without any barriers.

2. Cultural relevance: In Nigeria, walking is deeply ingrained in the culture. It is a common mode of transportation for many individuals especially in the countryside, where walking to nearby destinations is a way of life. Embracing walking as an exercise aligns well with existing cultural norms.

3. Cost-effective: With no need for expensive gym memberships or equipment, walking is a cost-effective exercise option for Nigerians. All that is required is a comfortable pair of walking shoes, which are readily available and affordable.

4. Climate suitability: Nigeria's climate is diverse, ranging from tropical in the south to arid in the north. Walking can be adapted to suit various weather conditions, making it a feasible exercise option year-round.

5. Natural scenery: Walking provides an opportunity for to connect with nature and enjoy the scenic landscapes while engaging in physical activity.

6. Social interaction: Walking can be a social activity, allowing you to walk with friends, family, or neighbours. This fosters a sense of community and support, making it a more enjoyable and sustainable exercise option.

7. Weight management: Given the increasing prevalence of obesity as a result of diet and lifestyle choices, walking offers a simple and effective means of weight management. It can be easily incorporated into daily routines, promoting regular physical activity and calorie burning.

8. Heart health: Nigeria, like many other countries, faces the challenge of heart-related health issues. Walking is an excellent cardiovascular exercise that can improve heart health, reduce the risk of heart disease, and lower blood pressure.

9. Stress reduction: With the fast-paced nature of modern life, stress has become a significant concern for many. Walking can serve as a stress-relief activity, promoting mental well-being and enhancing overall quality of life.

10. Sustainable lifestyle change: Sustainable lifestyle changes are vital for maintaining

long-term health and fitness. Walking is a practical and sustainable exercise option that can be easily integrated into daily routines, supporting a healthier lifestyle.

In conclusion, walking is a highly suitable exercise for Nigerians due to its accessibility, cost-effectiveness, and adaptability to the country's diverse climate and natural scenery.

Embracing walking as a regular form of exercise can not only contribute to better physical health but also foster a sense of community, reduce stress, and enhance overall well-being.

As Nigerians continue to prioritise their

health and fitness, walking stands as an ideal choice for promoting an active and fulfilling lifestyle.

Chapter 1:

Understanding the Concept of Weight Loss

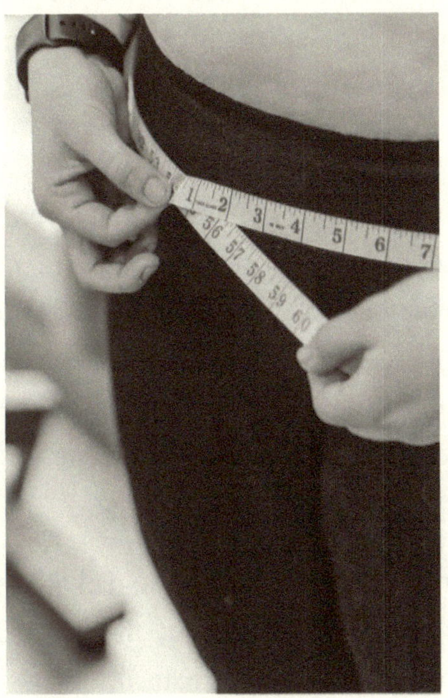

image from pexels.com

Weight loss is a fundamental concept in the realm of health and fitness, referring to the process of reducing body weight, predominantly through the loss of body fat. It involves creating a negative energy balance, where the calories expended by the body exceed the calories consumed through food and beverages. Understanding the concept of weight loss involves grasping the underlying principles, factors that influence it, and the importance of adopting a holistic approach to achieve sustainable and healthy results.

At its core, weight loss revolves around the simple principle of calorie balance. When the body consumes more calories than it expends, the excess energy is stored as fat, leading to weight gain. Conversely, when the body expends more calories than it consumes, it starts tapping into the fat stores for energy, resulting in weight loss.

It is crucial to understand that weight gain is not solely determined by the number of times you eat in a day. Instead, it is primarily influenced by the balance between your calorie intake and expenditure. If your daily calorie intake exceeds what you burn, the surplus will be stored as fat, leading to weight gain.

This clarification is essential for those who believe that eating only once a day will prevent weight gain, as it ultimately comes down to the total calorie balance. It's essential to be mindful of both the quantity and quality of the food you consume to maintain a healthy weight and overall well-being.

Several factors contribute to weight loss, and it is essential to consider them all to achieve success:

1. Diet: A balanced and nutritious diet plays a pivotal role in weight loss. Choosing nutrient-dense foods, controlling portion sizes, and being mindful of calorie intake are crucial components of an effective weight loss plan.

2. Physical activity: Regular exercise, including aerobic activities like walking, running, or swimming, as well

as strength training, helps burn calories, build lean muscle mass, and boost metabolism, contributing to weight loss.

3. Metabolism: Individual metabolic rate influences weight loss. Metabolism refers to the body's energy expenditure at rest. Some individuals have a higher metabolism and naturally burn more calories, while others have a slower metabolism, making weight loss a bit more challenging.

4. Genetics: Genetic factors can affect weight loss outcomes, as some individuals may be more predisposed to store or burn fat efficiently. However, genetics should not be considered an insurmountable barrier to weight loss; lifestyle changes can still have a significant impact. I fall within this category.

5. Hormones: Hormones play a crucial role in regulating appetite, hunger, and fat storage. Hormonal imbalances can

affect weight loss efforts and may require medical attention for proper management.

6. Behavior and lifestyle: Behavioral patterns, such as emotional eating, sedentary habits, and irregular sleep patterns, can hinder weight loss progress. Adopting healthy behaviours and lifestyle changes is vital for long-term success.

7. Certain medical conditions and medications: Certain medical conditions and medications can influence body weight. For instance, hypothyroidism, a condition where the thyroid is underactive, may lead to weight gain. Medications such as corticosteroids, antidepressants, and certain antipsychotics can also contribute to weight changes. Individuals experiencing unexplained weight fluctuations should consult with a healthcare professional to explore potential underlying medical causes.

It's essential to approach weight loss with a focus on overall health and well-being. Rapid or extreme weight loss methods, such as crash diets or fad diets, can be harmful to the body and often lead to unsustainable results. Healthy weight loss is gradual, aiming for a modest and steady reduction in body weight over time.

Additionally, weight loss should be accompanied by an emphasis on body composition rather than just the number on the scale. Building lean muscle through strength training can contribute to a toned and healthier physique while maintaining a stable weight.

Finally, it's essential to recognise that individual weight loss journeys may vary. Some people may experience rapid progress, while others may face plateaus or slower results. Patience, consistency, and perseverance are key to achieving sustainable weight loss and, more importantly, maintaining a healthy lifestyle in the long run.

Some Factors Affecting Weight Gain in Nigeria

Weight gain in Nigeria, as in any other country, is influenced by a combination of factors, including cultural, environmental, genetic, and lifestyle-related elements. Understanding these factors is essential in addressing the growing concern of obesity and promoting healthier lifestyles. Here are some of the key factors affecting weight gain in Nigeria:

1. Urbanisation and sedentary lifestyle: As Nigeria undergoes urbanisation, more people are leading sedentary lifestyles due to modern conveniences and technology. With increased screen time and decreased physical activity, the risk of weight gain rises.

2. Changing dietary habits: Traditional Nigerian diets were largely plant-based and locally sourced. However, with globalisation and increased access to processed and high-calorie foods, dietary habits have shifted towards more calorie-

dense options, leading to weight gain.

3. High caloric intake: Nigerian cuisine often includes calorie-rich dishes like jollof rice, fried plantains, starchy foods and swallows. However, consuming excessive calories without balancing it with physical activity can contribute to weight gain.

4. Lack of nutritional awareness: A lack of nutritional awareness and education can result in poor food choices and imbalanced diets, leading to overeating and weight gain.

5. Genetic predisposition: genetic factors can influence an individual's susceptibility to weight gain. Some people may be more prone to store excess calories as fat, making it challenging to maintain a healthy weight. Challenging but not unsurmountable.

6. Socioeconomic status: Low-income individuals may have limited access to nutritious foods, which can lead to

reliance on cheaper, calorie-dense options, mostly carbohydrates. A typical low income person can consume "Eba" in the morning, afternoon and night. In contrast, higher-income individuals may have greater access to a variety of foods and resources for healthier lifestyles.

7. Nutritious foods and fruits can really be expensive in many parts of the country.

8. Cultural norms: In some Nigerian cultures, being overweight is associated with wealth and prosperity, leading to a lack of concern about weight gain. Additionally, cultural festivities and celebrations often involve indulgent and calorie-rich foods. For us, food is a very important part of any celebration or festivities. We call it "ITEM 7"

9. Lack of physical activity facilities: Limited access to recreational facilities and safe outdoor spaces (especially in the cities) for physical activity can discourage exercise and contribute to weight gain.

10. Stress and emotional eating: Modern life in Nigeria can be stressful, and some individuals turn to food as a coping mechanism. Emotional eating, which involves eating to manage emotions rather than hunger, can lead to weight gain over time.

11. Medical conditions and medications: Certain medical conditions and medications can contribute to weight gain as a side effect or by affecting appetite and metabolism.

Addressing these factors requires a multi-faceted approach involving individuals, communities, healthcare providers, and policymakers. Promoting nutritional education, creating opportunities for physical activity, and raising awareness about the importance of maintaining a healthy weight are crucial steps in combating the issue of weight gain in Nigeria.

Encouraging a return to traditional diets rich in whole foods, coupled with regular physical activity, can help tackle the problem of obesity and promote healthier lifestyles across the country.

The Importance of Adopting a Healthy Lifestyle

Adopting a healthy lifestyle is one of the most significant investments we can make in ourselves, with far-reaching benefits that extend beyond physical health. It plays a pivotal role in enhancing our overall quality of life and longevity.

It involves making conscious choices that promote well-being, encompassing various aspects of life, including diet, exercise, mental health, and social connections.

Here are some key reasons why embracing a healthy lifestyle is crucial:

1. Physical health: A healthy lifestyle significantly reduces the risk of chronic diseases such as heart disease, diabetes, and obesity. Regular exercise, a balanced diet, and avoiding harmful habits like smoking contribute to better physical health and increase life expectancy.

2. Mental health: A healthy lifestyle has a profound impact on mental well-being. Regular physical activity releases endorphins, the "feel-good" hormones, reducing stress, anxiety, and depression. A nutritious diet and adequate sleep also play essential roles in maintaining optimal mental health.

3. Energy and vitality: By nourishing our bodies with nutritious foods and staying physically active, we can experience increased energy levels and overall vitality. This renewed energy positively impacts daily activities and enhances productivity.

4. Weight management: Adopting a healthy lifestyle promotes weight management by maintaining a balance between calorie intake and expenditure. It helps prevent weight gain and reduces the risk of obesity-related health issues.

5. Enhanced immune system: A healthy lifestyle supports a robust immune system, making us more resilient to

infections and illnesses.

6. Quality sleep: Healthy lifestyle practices contribute to better sleep quality and patterns, ensuring that we wake up refreshed and ready to face the day.

7. Cognitive function: Regular exercise and a healthy diet are associated with improved cognitive function, memory, and reduced risk of cognitive decline as we age.

8. Reduced risk of lifestyle-related diseases: By adopting healthy habits, such as not smoking, not consuming alcohol, and eating a balanced diet, we can significantly reduce the risk of lifestyle-related diseases and conditions.

9. Emotional well-being: A healthy lifestyle promotes emotional well-being by providing a sense of accomplishment and self-worth. Taking care of ourselves physically fosters a positive self-image and self-esteem.

10. Social connections: Engaging in physical activities, group fitness classes, or sports can lead to social interactions and foster a sense of community, which positively impacts mental health and reduces feelings of isolation.

11. Longevity: Research consistently shows that individuals who adopt healthy lifestyles tend to live longer with healthier lives compared to those who don't prioritise their well-being.

12. Positive role model: Embracing a healthy lifestyle not only benefits us but also sets a positive example for our friends, family, and future generations. Being a role model can inspire others to make healthier choices.

In conclusion, adopting a healthy lifestyle is not a quick fix but a lifelong commitment to nurturing our physical, mental, and emotional well-being. By prioritising regular exercise, nutritious eating, and positive habits, we can reap the countless benefits that contribute to a fulfilling and vibrant life. As we embrace a healthy lifestyle, we empower ourselves to live life to the fullest, becoming the best version of ourselves for the benefit of both our present and future selves.

Chapter 2

Let's Get Started

Assess Your Current Fitness Level

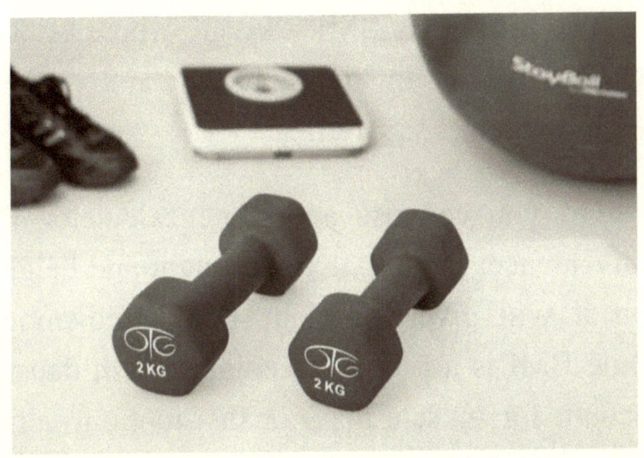

image from pexels.com

Assessing your current fitness level is essential before starting any exercise program, like walking for weight loss. It involves evaluating your past physical activity, cardiovascular endurance, strength, flexibility, balance, coordination, resting heart rate, body mass index (BMI), weight and body measurements. In addition, consider taking "before" photos. Visual documentation can be a powerful motivator and provide a tangible record of your progress.

Body Mass Index (BMI) Calculator Formula:

Body Mass Index is a simple calculation using a person's height and weight.

The formula is BMI = $kg/m2$ where kg is a person's weight in kilograms and m2 is their height in metres squared.

Or, you can use an online calculator for convenience. Just input your weight and height, and it will give you your BMI. Remember, while BMI is a useful screening tool, it doesn't account for muscle mass or distribution of fat, so it's advisable to interpret it alongside other health metrics.

Here's a general classification of BMI ranges:Underweight: BMI less than 18.5

Normal Weight: BMI between 18.5 and 24.9 Overweight: BMI between 25 and 29.9 Obese: BMI 30 or greater

Lastly, keep a fitness journal to track progress and set realistic goals.

Consulting a fitness professional or healthcare provider is advisable, especially if you have health concerns or are new to exercise.

Set Realistic And Achievable Goals

Weight loss is a journey, not a 100 meters dash. Setting realistic and achievable goals will set you up for success, help you stay motivated, and increase the likelihood of maintaining your weight loss in the long run. Unrealistic goals on the other hand, can lead to frustration, disappointment, and even the abandonment of your efforts.

Be aware that, embarking on a crash program or diet to lose weight may result in health consequences.

Focus on progress rather than perfection,

and embrace the positive changes you make along the way and celebrate the non-scale victories, for example, loss of a belt hole, previously tight clothes that now fit better etc.

Chapter 3

Walking Essentials

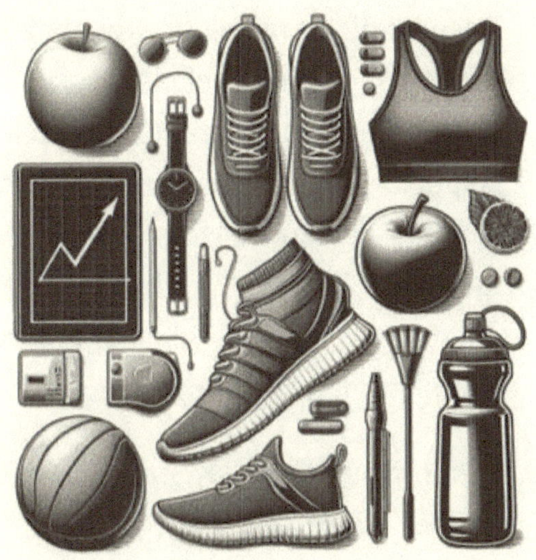

Created with Microsoft Bing AI Image Creator

A Correct Walking Posture

Maintaining the correct walking posture and technique not only enhance the effectiveness of your walking workouts but also promote overall joint and muscle health while minimisng the risk of injury.

Here are some tips to help you achieve the correct walking posture and technique:

1. Stand tall: Stand with your head held high, shoulders relaxed, and chest lifted. Engage your core muscles to support your spine and maintain a neutral posture. To engage your core muscles, imagine pulling your belly button in toward your spine while maintaining normal breathing.

2. Align your body: Keep your body in proper alignment while walking. Your ears, shoulders, hips, and ankles should be in a straight line, and your feet should be pointing forward.

3. Swing your arms: Bend your arms at a

90-degree angle and swing them naturally as you walk. The movement of your arms helps maintain balance and propels you forward.

4. Take comfortable strides: Take natural and comfortable strides, neither too short nor too long. Your feet should land softly with each step, rolling smoothly from heel to toe.

5. Heel-to-toe walking: Focus on a heel-to-toe walking motion. Land on your heel, roll through the ball of your foot, and push off with your toes. This rolling action allows for a more efficientstride.

6. Keep a brisk pace: Aim for a brisk walking pace that elevates your heart rate. You should beable to talk but feel slightly out of breath. Walking at a faster pace increases the calorie-burning potential.

7. Look ahead: Look forward, not down, to maintain good posture and be aware

of your surroundings. Keeping your gaze ahead also helps you walk in a straight line.

8. Keep your hips in check: Avoid swaying your hips from side to side. Keep them in line with your body's forward movement. Ladies, take note.

9. Wear proper footwear: Invest in comfortable and supportive walking shoes that fit well and provide adequate cushioning for your feet.

10. Warm-up and cool down: Warm up your muscles before starting your walk with gentle movements, and cool down with stretching exercises to prevent stiffness and injury.

11. Stay hydrated: Drink water before, during, and after your walk to stay hydrated, especially in hot or humid weather.

Practice these tips consistently, and over time, they will become second nature, allowing you to enjoy the full benefits of walking as a form of exercise.

If you have any specific concerns or health conditions, consider consulting a fitness professional or healthcare provider for personalised guidance.

Choosing The Right Walking Shoes

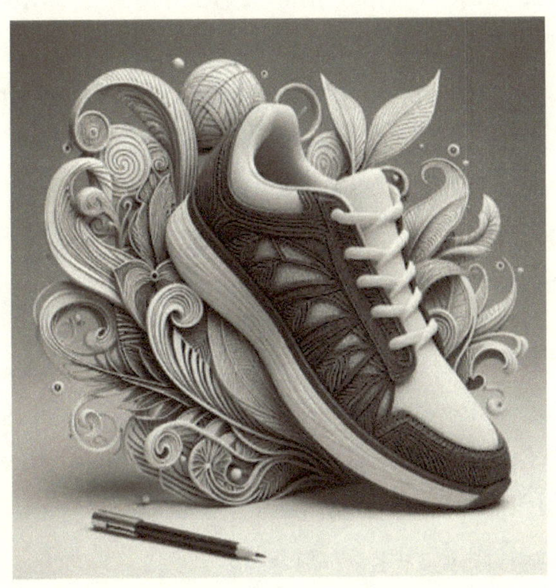

created with Microsoft Bing AI Image Creator

Selecting the appropriate walking shoes is of utmost importance to ensure a comfortable and injury-free walking journey. When I first began my consistent walking routine, I didn't pay much attention to wearing proper walking shoes. Instead, during walk at home sessions especially, I simply walked on the hard surface without any supportive footwear or a rug. Unfortunately, this led to discomfort and pains in my ankles, knees, and hips.

It quickly became evident that walking shoes are a crucial tool in maintaining an injury-free and enjoyable walking experience. Investing in the right pair of walking shoes can provide the necessary support, cushioning, and stability, reducing the impact on joints and preventing potential injuries.

Now, I prioritise wearing proper walking shoes whenever I head out for my walks or walking at home, knowing that they play a significant role in enhancing both my comfort and safety during every step.

Here are some key tips:

1. Proper fit: Ensure the shoes fit well with enough toe wiggle room and a

snug heel. Try them on with walking socks to get an accurate fit.

2. Arch support: Look for shoes with adequate arch support to prevent foot fatigue and discomfort during long walks.

3. Cushioning: Opt for shoes with sufficient cushioning in the heel and midsole to absorb impact and reduce strain on joints.

4. Breathability: Choose shoes made of breathable materials to keep your feet cool and dry during walks.

5. Flexibility: Check that the shoes have some flexibility in the forefoot to allow for a natural walking motion.

6. Grip: Look for shoes with a good rubber outsole for traction and stability, especially on different surfaces.

7. Weight: Select lightweight shoes to prevent excess fatigue during walks.

8. Activity-specific: Consider your walking terrain (pavement, trails, etc.) and choose shoes designed for that specific activity.

9. Try before buying: Always try on the shoes and walk around the store to ensure comfort and proper fit.

Remember that everyone's feet are different, so what works for one person may not work for another. Take your time to find the shoes that provide the best support and comfort for your individual needs.

There is however a time that walking shoes should be discarded and that is when you are grounding or earthing. (More about this later).

Safety Precautions For Outdoor Walking

Safety is paramount when engaging in outdoor walking not only to ensure a pleasant and injury-free experience but also to safeguard life amidst growing insecurities.

Here are some essential safety precautions to keep in mind:

1. Be visible: If walking during low-light conditions or at night, wear reflective clothing or accessories to make yourself visible to motorists and cyclists.

2. Choose safe routes: Select well-lit and well-maintained paths, sidewalks, or walking trails. Avoid walking on busy roads without sidewalks whenever possible.

3. Be aware of surroundings: Stay alert and aware of your surroundings. Avoid distractions from headphones or mobile devices that may prevent you from hearing approaching vehicles or potential hazards.

4. Cross streets Safely: Always use designated crosswalks and pedestrian crossings. Wait for traffic signals and look both ways before crossing the road.

5. Walk facing traffic: If walking on roads

without sidewalks, walk facing oncoming traffic to see vehicles approaching.

6. Dress appropriately: Wear weather-appropriate clothing, including proper footwear, to ensure comfort and protection during your walk.

7. Carry identification: Bring some form of identification, such as an ID card or a wristband with emergency contact information, in case of any unforeseen situations.

8. Walk with a friend or a group: Whenever possible, walk with a friend or a group, especially in unfamiliar or isolated areas.

9. Hydration: Carry a water bottle to stay hydrated, especially in hot weather.

10. Sunscreen and hat: Apply sunscreen and wear a hat to protect yourself from the sun's harmful rays during daytime walks.

11. Respect private property: Stick to public areas and avoid trespassing on private property.

12. Carry a mobile phone: Bring a fully charged mobile phone with you for emergencies or to call for assistance if needed.

By following these safety precautions, you can enjoy the benefits of outdoor walking while minimising potential risks and ensuring a safe and enjoyable experience.

Remember that safety should always be a priority, no matter where or when you walk.

Create A Walking Routine

Creating a walking routine is a great way to stay consistent and make walking a regular part of your daily life.

By creating a walking routine that suits your lifestyle and preferences, you'll find it easier to maintain consistency and make walking a healthy and enjoyable habit. As you progress, you can gradually increase the intensity and duration of your walks, reaping even more benefits from this simple yet effective form of exercise.

In addition, explore different walking routes to keep things interesting and prevent boredom. Walk in parks, neighbourhoods, or trails for variety.

How many Walking Steps per day is Ideal for Improved Health

The meta-analysis involving 15 studies and nearly 50,000 adults from four continents provides valuable insights into the optimal amount of daily walking steps for improved health and longevity.

A group of researchers studied almost 50,000 adults from different parts of the world for around seven years. They wanted to find out how many steps people should take each day for better health and a longer life, and if this number is different for different age groups.

They discovered that taking more steps each day is linked to a lower risk of early death. For people aged 60 and older, walking about 6,000 to 8,000 steps a day is enough for better health. For younger adults, around 8,000 to

10,000 steps a day is beneficial.

The researchers found that it's not just about walking faster; simply taking more steps is what matters most for a lower risk of death. Walking is a simple and effective way to improve health, and even a small increase in daily steps can make a difference.

So, the takeaway is that walking more each day, even if it's just a little bit more, can be really good for your health. For older adults, aim for about 6,000 to 8,000 steps a day, and for younger adults, around 8,000 to 10,000 steps a day is beneficial. Walking is an easy and accessible form of exercise that can help improve your well-being and longevity.

It is recommended that you wear a pedometer or download a fitness app to daily track your steps and progress.

Chapter 4:

Nutrition for Weight Loss

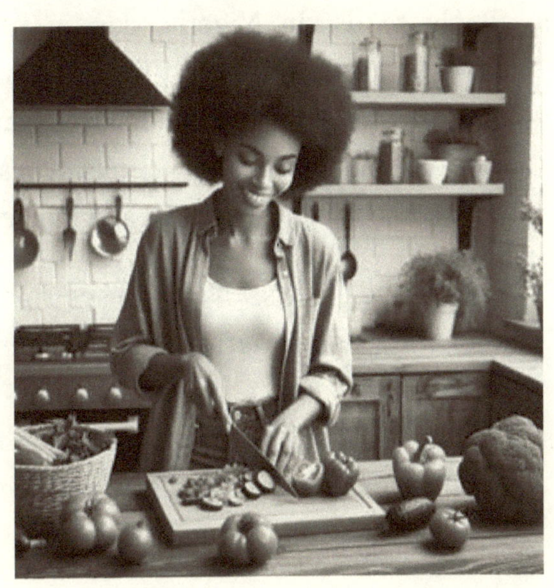

Understanding Nigerian dietary habits

Understanding Nigerian dietary habits is essential to appreciate the cultural significance of food and its role in daily life. Nigerian cuisine is rich and diverse, reflecting the country's various ethnic groups and regions. While dietary habits can vary among individuals and communities, some common characteristics are prevalent:

1. Staple foods: In Nigeria, certain foods serve as staple foods and form the basis of many meals. These include rice, yams, cassava, plantains, and various types of grains like millet, sorghum, and maize.

2. Soups and stews: Nigerian cuisine is known for its flavourful soups and stews, often made with a combination of vegetables, meat, fish, or poultry. Some popular examples include Egusi soup, Ogbono soup, and Efo riro.

3. Swallows: Swallows are starchy accompaniments to soups and stews. They are made by boiling starchy foods

like yams, cassava, or plantains and then pounding them into a smooth, stretchy consistency. Swallows are eaten by dipping them into the accompanying soup.

4. Meat and fish: Meat, especially beef, chicken, and goat, is a common protein source in Nigerian diets. Fish, both freshwater and seafood, is also widely consumed, particularly in coastal regions.

5. Spices and seasonings: Nigerian cuisine is known for its robust use of spices and seasonings, such as onions, garlic, ginger, and various local herbs and spices, which add depth and flavour to dishes.

6. Street Food: Street food is an integral part of Nigerian culinary culture. Hawkers sell a wide variety of snacks, such as puff-puff (deep-fried dough), suya (grilled meat skewers), and akara (fried bean cakes), which are popular among Nigerians.

7. Sweets and desserts: Desserts like chin chin (crunchy fried snacks), coconut candy, and puff-puff are enjoyed as treats and during celebrations.

8. Cultural significance: Food holds significant cultural importance in Nigeria, and traditional meals are often served during special occasions, festivals, and ceremonies, showcasing the country's rich cultural heritage.

9. Regional variations: Nigerian dietary habits vary across regions due to different agricultural practices and cultural influences. For example, the diet in the northern regions might include more grains and cereals, while coastal regions have a stronger emphasis on seafood.

10. Hydration: Alongside meals, Nigerians typically enjoy various beverages, including traditional drinks like palm wine, kunu (millet drink), and zobo (hibiscus tea), as well as soft drinks and water.

Understanding Nigerian dietary habits provides insights into the country's culture, history, and social practices. It highlights the importance of traditional foods, communal dining, and the significance of sharing meals with family and friends.

As Nigeria continues to modernise, traditional dietary habits are also evolving, with increased access to global cuisines and changes in lifestyle influencing food choices among its diversepopulation.

Healthy Food Choices For Weight Loss

Enjoy the rich flavours and diversity of Nigerian cuisine while incorporating healthier cooking methods and portion control to achieve your weight loss objectives. If you have specific dietary needs or health concerns, consider seeking guidance from a registered dietitian familiar with Nigerian cuisine.

Making healthy food choices is crucial for successful weight loss and overall well-being. Here are some nutritious options to support your weight loss goals:

1. Vegetables: Incorporate a variety of colourful vegetables into your meals. They are low in calories and high in essential nutrients, fiber, and antioxidants. Aim for leafy greens, broccoli, bell peppers, carrots, and tomatoes.

2. Fruits: Choose whole fruits as a natural source of sweetness and vitamins. Opt for fresh or frozen fruits over fruit juices or canned fruits with added sugars.

3. Lean proteins: Include lean protein sources in your diet to help build and maintain muscle while keeping you feeling full. Examples include skinless poultry, lean cuts of beef, fish, legumes, and beans.

4. Whole grains: Opt for whole grains like brown rice, quinoa, oats, and whole grain bread over refined grains. Whole grains provide more fiber and nutrients, keeping you satisfied for longer.

5. Healthy fats: Incorporate sources of healthy fats, such as avocados, nuts, seeds, and olive oil. These fats are beneficial for heart health and can help control hunger. Consider careful selection of your cooking oil, avoid saturated fats as much as you can. Most of what are tagged vegetable oil in our markets are saturated fats. Read labels.

6. Low-fat dairy: Choose low-fat or non-fat dairy products like yogurt, and cheese to reduce saturated fat intake.

7. Portion control: Be mindful of portion sizes to avoid overeating, even when consuming healthy foods.

8. Water: Stay hydrated by drinking plenty of water throughout the day. Sometimes thirst can be mistaken for hunger.

9. Limit added sugars: Reduce the intake of added sugars found in sugary drinks, sweets, and processed foods.

10. Mindful eating: Practice mindful eating

by paying attention to hunger and fullness cues, eating slowly, and savoring each bite.

11. Meal planning: Plan your meals and snacks ahead of time to avoid impulsive and unhealthy food choices.

12. Healthy snacks: Keep healthy snacks like fruit, or cut vegetables on hand for when hunger strikes between meals.

Remember, weight loss is not about deprivation but about making sustainable and healthier choices. Focus on nutrient-dense foods that provide nourishment while limiting highly processed and high-calorie options. Incorporating a balanced and varied diet, along with regular physical activity, is key to achieving and maintaining weight loss in the long run.

Balancing Macronutrients and Portion Control

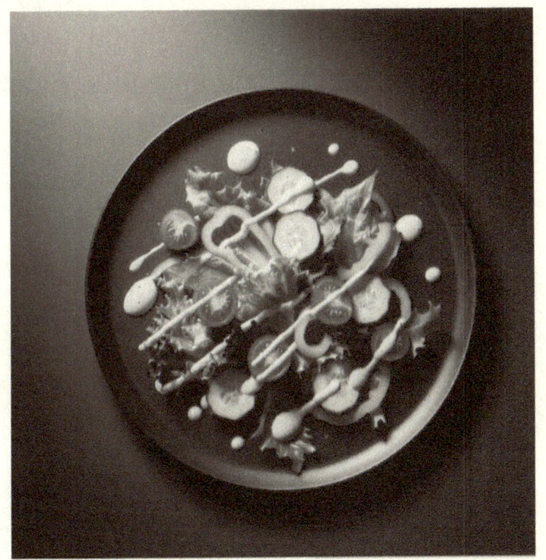

created with Microsoft Bing AI Image Creator

1. Understanding macronutrients:

  - Carbohydrates: Complex
    carbohydrates from Nigerian staples
    include rice, yams, plantains, and
    whole grains. These provide
    sustained energy and essential
    nutrients.

- Proteins: Include lean protein sources like chicken, fish, beans, and local legumes (e.g., cowpeas, lentils). Proteins support muscle maintenance and growth.

- Fats: Choose healthy fats from sources like palm oil, groundnut oil, avocados, and nuts. These fats are important for overall health and satiety.

2. Portion control:

- Be mindful: Listen to your body's hunger and fullness signals. Eat slowly and stop when you feel satisfied, not overly full.

- Use a small sized plate.

- Divide Your Plate: Mentally divide your plate into portions for soups, stews, or swallow (carbohydrates), proteins, and vegetables. Serve appropriate amounts of each.

- Avoid wastage: Prepare and serve

portions that are suitable for your needs to avoid food wastage.

3. Balancing meals:

- Include vegetables: Incorporate a variety of Nigerian vegetables like ugwu, waterleaf, spinach, and okra in your meals for added nutrients and fiber.

4. Snack wisely:

- Opt for local snacks: Choose healthy Nigerian snacks like roasted plantains, groundnuts, or kuli-kuli (groundnut cakes).

- Mind portion sizes: Control portions when snacking to prevent excessive calorie intake.

5. Read labels:

- Select healthier brands: When buying packaged foods, consider brands with familiar ingredients and nutritional information.

- Watch serving sizes: Be aware of serving sizes to avoid overeating processed snacks.

6. Personalise your plan:

- Tailor your eating plan to include foods and dishes that suit your taste and culturalpreferences.

- Seek local advice: Consult with a registered dietitian familiar with Nigerian cuisine for personalised guidance.

Embracing and navigating locally available foods and local dietary practices can be an integral part of a healthy weight loss journey.

By balancing macronutrients and controlling portions, individuals can create sustainable eating habits for long-term well-being.

Chapter 5

Overcoming Challenges

Dealing with Time Constraints in Walking for Weight Loss

Dealing with time constraints while walking for weight loss requires creativity and commitment. Here are some strategies to overcome this challenge:

1. Short walks: Incorporate short walks into your daily routine, even if it's just for 10-15 minutes. Consistency is key.

2. Prioritise: Make walking a priority and treat it as an essential appointment with yourself.

3. Early mornings: Consider waking up a

bit earlier to fit in a morning walk before the day gets busy.

4. Lunch break: Use your lunch break for a quick walk, even if it's just around your office building or neighbourhood.

5. Family walks: Involve your family in walking, turning it into a bonding activity.

6. Multitask: Combine walking with other tasks, like walking to nearby places instead of driving.

7. Home workouts: On busy days and unfavourable weather conditions, try home workouts or bodyweight exercises to stay active.

8. Track progress: Keep a walking journal or use a fitness app to monitor your progress and stay motivated.

9. Be realistic: Set achievable walking goals that fit your schedule, and don't be too hard on yourself if you miss a day.

By being resourceful and creative with your time, you can successfully incorporate walking into your daily routine, making it a powerful tool for weight loss and overall health.

Walking During Unfavourable Weather Conditions

Walking during unfavourable weather conditions requires adaptability and consideration for safety.

Here are some tips to make the most of your walking routine despite challenging weather:

1. Rainy days:

   - Wear waterproof gear: Invest in a good-quality waterproof jacket, shoes, and an umbrella to stay dry during light rain.

   - Choose covered routes: Opt for walking paths with some form of cover, like tree-lined streets or pathways with overhead bridges.

- Embrace the rain: If the rain isn't too heavy, consider walking in it with appropriate rain gear. Walking in the rain can be refreshing and invigorating.

2. Hot weather:

   - Walk early or late: Plan your walks during the cooler parts of the day, such as early mornings or late evenings.

   - Stay hydrated: Carry a water bottle and drink plenty of fluids to stay hydrated during hot weather walks.

   - Dress appropriately: Wear loose, breathable clothing and a hat to protect yourself from the sun.

3. Cold weather:

   - Layer up: Dress in layers to stay warm. Start with a moisture-wicking base layer, add an insulating layer, and finish with a windproof outer layer.

- Protect extremities: Wear gloves, a scarf, and a beanie to keep your hands, neck, and head warm.

- Warm up indoors: Do a quick warm-up indoors before heading out into the cold to prevent injury.

4. Thunderstorms:

- Safety first: Avoid walking outdoors during thunderstorms or when lightning is present. Seek shelter until the storm passes.

- Plan indoor activities: Have backup indoor exercises or activities ready for stormy days.

5. Air pollution:

- Check air quality: Be mindful of air pollution levels, especially in urban areas. If air quality is poor, consider indoor exercise options.

6. Extreme weather:

- Know your limits: In cases of extreme weather like severe cold, prioritise your safety and consider alternative indoor exercises.

- Listen to your body: Pay attention to how your body feels during walks and adjust your pace or distance accordingly.

Remember, safety comes first. Always consider the weather conditions and how they may affect your health and well-being.

Adapt your walking routine to accommodate unfavorable weather, and don't hesitate to explore indoor exercise options when needed. Staying flexible and making wise choices will ensure you can maintain your walking routine year-round, regardless of the weather.

Managing Muscle Soreness And Injury Prevention

It is normal to experience some muscle soreness, especially when starting a new exercise routine including walking for weight loss. However, if soreness is severe or persists for an extended period, it's essential to listen to your body and seek medical advice if needed.

Prioritising injury prevention and recovery will help you enjoy the benefits of walking for weight loss safely and effectively.

Here are some tips to help you stay safe and minimise muscle soreness:

1. Warm-up and cool down: Always start your walking sessions with a 5-10 minute warm-up of light walking or gentle stretching to prepare your muscles for activity. Similarly, end your walks with a cool-down to gradually lower your heart rate and stretch your muscles.

2. Proper walking form: Pay attention to your walking posture and technique.

Maintain an upright posture, swing your arms naturally, and take comfortable strides. Avoid overstriding or slouching.

3. Gradual progression: If you're new to walking or increasing your walking distance, do so gradually. Sudden intense workouts can lead to muscle soreness and injuries.

4. Listen to your Body: Pay attention to any signs of discomfort or pain during or after walking. If you experience persistent pain, stop and rest. If the pain persists, seek medical advice.

5. Stretching: Incorporate stretching exercises for major muscle groups, such as calves, hamstrings, quadriceps, and hip flexors, after your walks. Stretching helps improve flexibility and reduce muscle tightness.

6. Strength training: Include strength training exercises in your routine. Strengthening the muscles around your joints can help prevent injuries and

improve overall stability.

7. Footwear: Wear comfortable and supportive walking shoes that fit well. Replace worn-out shoes to avoid potential foot and ankle problems. Avoid previously owned walking shoes (known locally as second hand) as much as possible or do a proper evaluation if you must buy one.

8. Hydration: Stay well-hydrated during walks, especially in hot weather, to prevent muscle cramps and fatigue.

9. Rest days: Allow your body sufficient time to recover between walking sessions. Rest days are essential for muscle repair and preventing overuse injuries.

10. Cross-training: Include other low-impact exercises like swimming or cycling to give your walking muscles a break while still maintaining your fitness level.

11. Massage and foam rolling: Consider

using a foam roller or getting regular massages to relieve muscle soreness and improve recovery.

12. Injury prevention exercises: Incorporate exercises that target specific areas prone to injuries, such as ankle circles and calf raises, to enhance joint stability.

Chapter 6

Maximising Results

Combining Walking with Strength Training

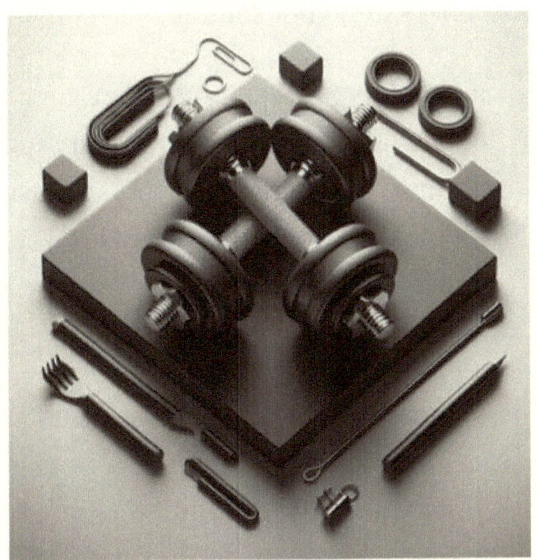

created with Microsoft Bing AI Image Creator

Walking is an inexpensive exercise and affordable for most, if not all, except for individuals with certain health conditions. Personally, walking works well for me both for controlling weight and maintaining overall health.

Walking however, with strength training can be a powerful approach to enhance fitness, promote weight loss, and improve overall health.

Here is how you can effectively integrate both exercises into your routine:

1. Schedule your walkouts: Plan your week to include both walking and strength training sessions. Aim for at least 150 minutes of moderate-intensity aerobic activity (like walking) and two or more days of strength training per week.

2. Alternate days: On alternate days, perform strength training exercises to allow your muscles time to recover from the intense workout.

3. Warm-up: Before each strength training session, warm up with a 5-10 minute brisk walk to increase blood flow and prepare your muscles for exercise.

4. Full-body strength training: Focus on compound exercises that target multiple muscle groups simultaneously, such as squats, lunges, push-ups, and rows. This will maximise the efficiency of your workouts.

5. Body-weight rxercises: If you don't have access to weights, use your body weight for resistance in exercises like planks, push-ups, and bodyweight squats.

6. Resistance training: Incorporate resistance bands or dumbbells to add intensity to your strength training routine. Gradually increase the resistance as you get stronger.

7. Recovery: Allow hours of rest between strength training sessions targeting the same muscle groups.

8. Balance and core: Include exercises that improve balance and core strength, such as single-leg squats, bridges, and plank variations.

9. Post-walk stretching: After your walks, perform stretching exercises to improve flexibility and reduce muscle tightness.

10. Progression: Gradually increase the intensity of your strength training workouts by adding more sets, repetitions, or weight.

11. Listen to your body: Pay attention to how your body responds to the combined workouts. If you feel overly fatigued or experience pain, modify your routine or take a rest day.

12. Seek professional guidance: If you're new to strength training, consider working with a fitness trainer to ensure proper form and technique.

Combining walking with strength training creates a well-rounded exercise program that targets cardiovascular fitness, muscle strength, and flexibility. Not only will this approach aid in weightloss and muscle toning, but it will also improve your overall fitness level and support a healthy lifestyle. As with any exercise routine, consistency and patience are key to seeing long-term results.

Chapter 7

Cultivating A Positive Mindset For Sustainable Weight Loss

Cultivating a positive mindset is vital for long-term and sustainable weight loss. The path to achieving and maintaining a healthy weight may present challenges, but with the right mindset, it becomes more manageable and even enjoyable.

For me, discovering my WHY has been instrumental in overcoming obstacles along my weight loss journey. My WHY serves as the core of my motivation and keeps me focused on my goals.

To sustain a compelling WHY, it must go

beyond pleasing others and instead prioritise the personal benefits of weight loss. Making myself the primary beneficiary of the positive outcomes has been a key factor in maintaining my commitment to the process.

Here are some tips to help you foster a positive mindset for long-term success:

1. Set realistic goals: Start by setting achievable and realistic weight loss goals. Break them down into smaller milestones, celebrating each achievement along the way.

2. Focus on progress, not perfection: Understand that weight loss is a gradual process, and setbacks may happen. Instead of fixating on perfection, celebrate your progress and the positive changes you've made.

3. Practice self-compassion: Be kind to yourself and avoid self-criticism. It's enough that people who do not understand your struggles with weight loss make unkind comments, you must

decide not to allow such comments set you back and make you to despise yourself. Treat yourself with the same understanding and support you would offer a friend on their weight loss journey.

4. Embrace positivity: Surround yourself with positive influences, whether it's supportive friends, inspirational books, or uplifting affirmations. A positive environment can fuel your motivation.

5. Visualise Success: Imagine yourself reaching your weight loss goals and living a healthier life. Visualisation can reinforce your commitment and determination.

6. Focus on non-scale victories: Recognise that success is not solely measured by the numbers on the scale. Celebrate non-scale victories, such as increased energy, improved mood, or better sleep.

7. Practice Mindful Eating: Pay attention to your body's hunger and fullness cues, and

savour each bite. Mindful eating helps you build a healthier relationship with food.

8. Positive affirmations: Use positive affirmations daily to boost your confidence and belief in yourself. Remind yourself that you are capable of achieving your goals.

9. Seek support: Surround yourself with a support network of friends, family, or a weight loss group. Having people who understand and encourage your journey can be incredibly motivating.

10. Focus on health, not just appearance: Shift your focus from solely wanting to change your appearance to prioritising your overall health and well-being. This mindset makes weight loss a positive step towards better health.

11. Learn from setbacks: View setbacks as learning opportunities rather than failures. Identify what triggered the setback and use it to develop strategies

for future success.

12. Be Patient: Sustainable weight loss takes time. Embrace the journey, knowing that slow and steady progress is more likely to lead to lasting results.

By nurturing a positive mindset, you'll build resilience and determination to overcome challenges that may arise during your weight loss journey. A positive outlook can make the process more enjoyable and sustainable, ultimately leading to a healthier and happier lifestyle. Remember, every step forward, no matter how small, brings you closer to your goals.

Conclusion:

In conclusion, "Walk It Out: A Walking For Weight Loss Guide for Nigerians" emphasises the incredible benefits of walking as a sustainable and effective exercise for achieving weight loss and overall health. Throughout this guide, we have explored essential topics tailored to the Nigerian audience, aiming to inspire and support you on your weight loss journey. Let's recap the key points:

1. Benefits of walking for weight loss: Walking is a simple yet powerful exercise that aids in burning calories, improving cardiovascular health, and boosting overall well-being.

2. Why walking is suitable for Nigerians: Walking is accessible, cost-effective, and culturally relevant for Nigerians, making it an ideal exercise for people of all ages.

3. Understanding weight loss: Weight loss is a gradual process that involves a combination of regular exercise, healthy eating, and lifestyle changes.

4. Factors affecting weight gain in Nigeria: Recognise the cultural, environmental, and dietary factors that contribute to weight gain in Nigeria to make informed choices.

5. Importance of qdopting a healthy lifestyle: Embrace a balanced and healthy

lifestyle to achieve sustainable weight
loss and overall wellness.

6. Assessing your current fitness Level:
   Understanding your starting point helps
   set realistic weight loss goals and ensures
   a safe exercise program.

7. Setting realistic weight loss goals: Break
   down your goals into achievable
   milestones to maintain motivation and
   track progress.

8. Correct walking posture and technique:
   Mastering the right walking form
   enhances the effectiveness of your walks
   and reduces the risk of injury.

9. Choosing the right walking shoes: Invest
   in comfortable and supportive shoes to
   make your walking experience enjoyable
   and safe.

10. Safety precautions for outdoor walking:
    Be mindful of safety measures, especially
    during unfavourable weather conditions,
    to prevent accidents and discomfort.

11. Creating a walking routine: Design a personalised walking program that suits your schedule and fitness level, and incorporate interval training for increased effectiveness.

12. Nutrition for weight loss: Understand Nigerian dietary habits and make healthy food choices while balancing macronutrients and practicing portion control.

13. Managing muscle soreness and injury Prevention: Prioritise warm-ups, cool-downs, and proper form to reduce muscle soreness and lower the risk of injuries.

14. Cultivating a positive mindset: Embrace a positive outlook, set realistic expectations, and focus on non-scale victories to support long-term weight loss success.

15. Boosting metabolism and burning more calories: Incorporate strength training, HIIT, and lifestyle habits that enhance metabolism and calorie burn.

Remember, sustainable weight loss is a journey that requires dedication, patience, and self-compassion. As you embark on this path, celebrate each step forward and learn from

setbacks. Focus on the long-term benefits of a healthier lifestyle, and always consult healthcare professionals for personalised guidance.

With the right mindset, commitment, and support, you have the power to transform your life through walking and embrace a healthier, happier you.

Start your journey now and remember that each step you take brings you closer to your goals. Wishing you success on your weight loss journey!

Final Tips for Success on Your Weight Loss Journey:

1. Stay consistent: Consistency is key to achieving lasting results. Make walking and healthy eating habits a regular part of your lifestyle.

2. Be patient and persistent: Sustainable weight loss takes time. Stay committed to your goals, even during challenging times.

3. Track your progress: Keep a journal or use a fitness app to monitor your walking sessions, nutrition, and any changes in your body. Seeing your progress can be motivating.

4. Celebrate non-scale victories: Celebrate the positive changes beyond the numbers on the scale, such as increased energy, improved mood, or better sleep.

5. Focus on health, Not perfection: Aim for overall health and well-being rather than striving for a perfect body. Your worth is not defined by a number.

6. Embrace setbacks as Learning Opportunities: If you face setbacks, view them as opportunities to learn and grow. Stay resilient and get back on track.

7. Seek support and accountability: Share

your goals with friends, family, or join a weight loss group for support and encouragement.

8. Balance your life: Take care of your physical, mental, and emotional health. Balance your weight loss efforts with self-care and relaxation.

9. Stay educated: Stay updated on nutrition and exercise trends. Knowledge empowers you to make informed decisions.

10. Don't compare yourself to others: Your journey is unique. Focus on your progress, and avoid comparing yourself to others.

11. Practice mindfulness: Be mindful of your eating habits, emotions, and responses. Mindfulness can help you make healthier choices.

12. Reward Yourself: Celebrate your achievements with non-food rewards, like treating yourself to a spa day or a

new workout outfit.

13. Never Give Up: Embrace challenges as opportunities to grow stronger. If you stumble, dust yourself off and keep moving forward.

14. Trust the process: Trust that the small steps you take each day will lead to significant and lasting changes over time.

15. Be kind to yourself: Show yourself kindness and self-compassion throughout your weight loss journey. You deserve to be your biggest cheerleader.

Remember, your weight loss journey is about improving your health and well-being, not achieving perfection. Focus on progress, take one step at a time, and embrace the positive changes along the way. You have the power to create a healthier and happier life. Trust in yourself, stay motivated, and keep your eyes on the long-term benefits of a healthier lifestyle. With determination and self-belief, success is within reach. Cheers!

Appendix 1

Grounding or Earthing

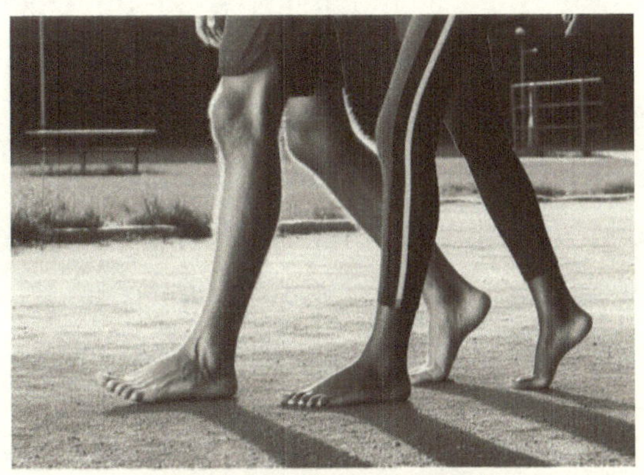

Walking Barefooted
created with Microsoft Bing AI Image Creator

Grounding, also known as earthing, is a practice that involves connecting with the Earth's surface to receive its natural electrical charge. This process allows us to harmonize with the Earth's energy and potentially gain health benefits.

In our modern lives, we often spend much of our time indoors or wearing shoes with insulating soles, which can create a disconnect from the Earth's energy. However, proponents of grounding believe that direct contact with the Earth's surface can restore this balance and positively impact our well-being.

The concept of grounding is based on the idea that the Earth carries a subtle electrical charge due to its interaction with the sun and other celestial bodies. When we make direct contact with the Earth through our skin or feet, we can absorb this electrical charge, which is believed to have antioxidant and anti-inflammatory effects on our bodies.

Advocates of grounding claim that it can:

1. Reduce inflammation: Grounding is thought to neutralise excess positive electrons in the body, which are associated with inflammation. By doing so, it may help alleviate chronic inflammatory conditions.

2. Improve sleep: Some people report improved sleep quality after practicing grounding. This may be attributed to its

potential stress-reducing and cortisol-balancing effects.

3. Enhance energy and vitality: Grounding is believed to increase feelings of vitality and energy by promoting a balanced electrical state in the body.

4. Alleviate pain: Grounding has been associated with pain reduction and improved muscle recovery, possibly due to its impact on inflammation and stress reduction.

5. Improve circulation: It is suggested that grounding may improve blood flow and circulation, benefiting cardiovascular health.

Grounding can be done in various ways, such as walking barefoot on natural surfaces like grass, soil, sand, or even wet surfaces like a beach. Some people also use grounding mats, sheets, or footwear that are designed to conduct the Earth's energy.

Overall, grounding is a simple and natural

practice that encourages us to reconnect with the Earth and embrace the potential benefits it may offer for our physical and emotional well-being.

Appendix 2

Walking Resources

Here are some walking resources to help you get started or enhance your walking routine:

1. Walking apps: There are several mobile apps designed to track your walking progress, and offer personalised training plans. Some popular apps include:

   - Pedometer: Counts your steps and helps you set daily step goals.

   - Google Fit.

2. Online walking Communities: Joining online walking communities can provide support, motivation, and tips from like-minded individuals.

3. YouTube walking workouts: Search for walking workout videos on YouTube. There are various channels offering guided walking workouts of different lengths and intensity levels. These videos can add variety to your routine and keep you engaged. My favourites are Leslie Sansone (walk at home) and Paul Eugene.

4. Walking challenges: Participate in walking challenges to keep yourself motivated. You can find challenges on fitness apps, online communities, or create your own with friends and family.

5. Local walking groups: Look for walking groups or clubs in your area. Joining a local walking group can provide social support, accountability, and the opportunity to explore new walking routes together.

6. Walking gear and accessories: Invest in comfortable walking shoes, moisture-wicking clothing, and a good quality water bottle to stay hydrated during your

walks.

7. Books on walking: Consider reading
   books that focus on walking for health
   and fitness.

8. Safety tips: Educate yourself on safety
   tips for walking, especially if you plan to
   walk outdoors or during specific weather
   conditions. Always walk in well-lit areas,
   use reflective gear in low-light situations,
   and carry a phone for emergencies.

Remember to consult with a healthcare
professional before starting any new exercise
routine, especially if you have any health
concerns or medical conditions. Enjoy your
walking journey and have fun exploring the
benefits of this simple yet effective form of
exercise!

Appendix 3

Seven Days Food Timetable for Weight Loss (with Nigerian Food)

This 7-day food timetable is tailored for Nigerians, featuring popular and nutritious Nigerian dishes. It provides a balanced mix of proteins, healthy fats, and carbohydrates while staying within a daily calorie intake of 1500 calories. As always, individual preferences and dietary restrictions can be considered when choosing specific food items and portion sizes. Remember to stay hydrated, practice portion control, and engage in regular physical activity for the best weight loss results.

Day 1:

- Breakfast: Moi Moi (steamed bean pudding) with a side of sliced cucumber (250 calories).

- Snack: Watermelon slices (50 calories).

- Lunch: Grilled chicken with jollof rice and mixed vegetables (400 calories).

- Snack: Handful of peanuts (100 calories).

- Dinner: Efo Riro (spinach stew) with baked fish and boiled plantains (600 calories).

- Total: 1400 calories.

Day 2:

- Breakfast: Akara (bean cake) with a side of garden egg slices (250 calories).

- Snack: Orange segments (50

calories).

- Lunch: Okra soup with chicken and a side of amala (yam flour) (400 calories).

- Snack: Sliced pineapple (100 calories).

- Dinner: Grilled tilapia with steamed vegetables and boiled yam (600 calories).

- Total: 1400 calories.

Day 3:

- Breakfast: Oats porridge with skimmed milk, diced apples, and a sprinkle of cinnamon (300 calories).

- Snack: Guava slices (50 calories).

- Lunch: Vegetable stir-fry with tofu and a side of boiled plantains (400 calories).

- Snack: Handful of cashew nuts (100 calories).

- Dinner: Moi Moi (steamed bean pudding) with a side of coleslaw (600 calories).

- Total: 1450 calories.

Day 4:

- Breakfast: Pap (ogi) with a handful of groundnuts (250 calories).

- Snack: Sliced cucumber with a dash of lemon juice (50 calories).

- Lunch: Grilled chicken with cabbage salad (400 calories).

- Snack: Mango slices (100 calories).

- Dinner: Efo Riro (spinach stew) with grilled tilapia and a side of boiled rice (600 calories).

- Total: 1400 calories.

Day 5:

- Breakfast: Moi Moi (steamed bean pudding) with diced avocado (250 calories).

- Snack: Watermelon cubes (50 calories).

- Lunch: Vegetable soup with goat meat and a side of pounded yam (400 calories).

- Snack: Handful of roasted groundnuts (100 calories).

- Dinner: Grilled mackerel with coleslaw and boiled plantains (600 calories).

- Total: 1400 calories.

Day 6:

- Breakfast: Boiled plantains with egg stew (250 calories).

- Snack: Sliced pineapple (50 calories).

- Lunch: Grilled chicken with jollof rice and mixed vegetables (400 calories).

- Snack: Handful of tiger nuts (100 calories).

- Dinner: Okra soup with fish and a side of eba (cassava flour) (600 calories).

- Total: 1400 calories.

Day 7:

- Breakfast: Vegetable omelette with whole wheat bread (250 calories).

- Snack: Guava slices (50 calories).

- Lunch: Moi Moi (steamed bean pudding) with a side of sliced cucumbers and tomatoes (400 calories).

- Snack: Handful of roasted peanuts (100 calories).

- Dinner: Grilled tilapia with vegetable stir-fry and boiled yam (600 calories).

- Total: 1400 calories.

Recommended Health Recovery & Weight Loss Protocol

If being overweight is already having a negative impact on your health, consider this protocol which is adapted from Dr Brooke Goldner's book, 'Goodbye Lupus'.

Program Duration - 6 Weeks (can be extended to accommodate better result)

1. No animal protein

2. Take prescribed smoothie throughout the day.

3. Adopt salad with healthy dressing as meals. If not able to do this, eat only once a day and be conscious of portion control. The smoothie is very filling.

4. If you have to eat cooked food, avoid oil except flaxseed oil, chia seed oil or hempseed oil. Consider cooking without oil for the six weeks.

5. Drink at least 3 litres of water daily

6. Take quarter teaspoon of Iodized salt daily

7. Supplement Vit B12

8. Exercise for at least 30 minutes daily

9. Get adequate sleep, not less than 7 hours daily.

Smoothie Recipe

1. Cruciferous vegetables - 1 pound or 0.454kg

2. Flax seeds or Chia seeds - half cup (standard measurement) or 3 tablespoons of Flaxseed oil.

3. Fruits (banana, pineapple, mangoes etc) in moderation. Be honest with yourself when adding fruits in this protocol, if too much, result may not be quick.

Method

1. Clean vegetables and put in blender.

2. Add water to the level of the vegetable in the blender

3. Add half cup of flax seeds or Chia seeds.

4. Fill up with banana, pineapple and mangoes or any fruit available. Addition of fruits is to enhance the taste and make a rich smoothie. It is optional.

The fruit is solely for taste. Faster result is achieved without the fruits

1. Blend until it's very smooth.

Drink throughout the day not at once.

Note

Clean your vegetables very well under running water but preferably with vinegar.

If your blender is not high power, blend your flaxseeds or Chia seeds in the dry part of your blender till smooth before putting it in the wet blender with the vegetable.

Don't freeze your vegetables but your fruits can be preserved in the fridge or freezer. You can use ginger and lemon in your smoothie and salad as preferred.

List of cruciferous vegetables for this protocol.

(You can stick to one or combine).

You must use at least one pound (1lb) or about half kg (0.454) daily for the smoothie.

They include:

- Arugula Bok choy

- Broccoli Broccoli rabe Broccoli romanesco Brussel sproutsCabbage

- Cauliflower Chinese broccoli Chinese cabbage Collard greens Daikon

- Garden cress HorseradishKale

- Kohlrabi Komatsuna Land cress

Mizuna

- Mustard – seeds and leavesRadish

- RutabagaTatsoi

- Turnips – root and greensWasabi

- Watercress.

- Cabbage is an available and affordable choice in Nigeria for everyone.

Sample Weight Loss Drinks

In Nigeria, there are various weight loss drinks that can be easily accessed and incorporated into your diet. Here are some popular ones:

1. Green tea: Green tea is rich in antioxidants and can help boost metabolism, making it a popular choice for weight loss. You can find green tea bags or loose leaves in supermarkets and open markets.

2. Hibiscus tea (Zobo): Hibiscus tea, also known as Zobo, is a flavourful and refreshing drink that can aid in weight management. It may help reduce water retention and has potential appetite-suppressing properties. This is recommended without added sugar.

3. Lemon water: Simple and effective, lemon water can be easily made by squeezing fresh lemon juice into a glass of water. Lemon is believed to promote digestion and detoxification, making it a popular choice for weight loss.

4. Cinnamon tea: Cinnamon has been shown to regulate blood sugar levels and improve insulin sensitivity, which can be helpful for weight management. Boil cinnamon sticks in water to make a soothing and fragrant tea.

5. Moringa tea: Moringa leaves are packed with nutrients and antioxidants. Drinking moringa tea can help boost energy levels and support weight loss efforts.

6. Ginger tea: Ginger has anti-inflammatory properties and can aid in digestion. Ginger tea is easy to make by steeping fresh ginger slices in hot water.

7. Bitter leaf juice: Bitter leaf juice is believed to have detoxifying properties and can help with digestion.

8. Apple Cider Vinegar (ACV) drink: Although not a traditional Nigerian beverage, apple cider vinegar is becoming more widely available. Mix one tablespoon of ACV with water and a bit of honey to make a weight loss tonic.

Remember that while these drinks can complement a healthy weight loss plan, they are not magic solutions. For effective and sustainable weight loss, it's essential to combine these drinks with a balanced diet, regular physical activity, and a healthy lifestyle. Additionally, consult with a healthcare professional before making significant changes to your diet, especially if you have any underlying health conditions.

Sample Fat Burning Recipes

1. Green tea and mint infusion:

    -   1 green tea bag or 1 teaspoon of loose green tea leaves

    -   1 handful of fresh mint leaves

    -   1 cup of boiling water

Steep the green tea bag or leaves in boiling water for 3-5 minutes. Add the fresh mint leaves and let it infuse for another 2-3 minutes. Strain the mixture and enjoy a refreshing fat-burning drink.

2. Hibiscus and ginger detox drink:

    -   2 tablespoons of dried hibiscus (Zobo) leaves or petals

    -   1-inch piece of fresh ginger, thinly sliced

    -   1 liter of water

    -   Optional: Honey or natural sweetener to taste

In a pot, bring the water to a boil and add the hibiscus leaves and ginger slices. Let it simmer for 10-15 minutes. Remove from heat and allow it to cool. Add honey or natural sweetener if desired. This drink is known for its detoxifying and metabolism-boosting properties.

3. Lemon and cucumber slimming water:

- 1 lemon, thinly sliced

- 1/2 cucumber, thinly sliced

- 1 liter of water

- Optional: A few sprigs of fresh mint for added flavour

Add the lemon and cucumber slices to one litre of water. If desired, add some fresh mint leaves. Let it infuse in the refrigerator for at least 2 hours before drinking. This hydrating drink can help with bloating and boost metabolism.

4. Ginger and turmeric metabolism

booster:

- 1-inch piece of fresh ginger, grated or thinly sliced

- 1/2 teaspoon of ground turmeric or 1-inch piece of fresh turmeric, grated

- Juice of 1 lemon

- 1 liter of water

- Optional: natural sweetener to taste

In one litre of water, combine the ginger, turmeric, and lemon juice. Add the water and let it infuse for a few hours. Sweeten with honey if desired. Ginger and turmeric are known for their metabolism-boosting and anti-inflammatory properties.

5. Pineapple and mint fat burner:

- 1 cup of fresh pineapple chunks

- 1 handful of fresh mint leaves

- 1 liter of water

- Optional: A dash of cayenne pepper for an extra kick

Blend the pineapple chunks and fresh mint leaves with water until smooth. Strain the mixture if desired, and add a dash of cayenne pepper for added fat-burning benefits. Enjoy this tropical and refreshing fat-burning drink.

6. Chia seed and lemon detox drink:

- 1 tablespoon chia seeds

- Juice of 1 lemon

- 1 bananaor any other fruit of choice (optional for sweetness)

- 1 liter of water

In a glass, mix the chia seeds with water and let it sit for 10 minutes until they form a gel-like consistency. Add the lemon juice and fruit (if using) and stir well. Chia seeds are rich in fiber and can help you feel fuller for longer, while lemon aids digestion and detoxification.

7. Fenugreek and cinnamon metabolism

booster:

- 1 teaspoon fenugreek seeds

- 1/2 teaspoon ground cinnamon

- 1 liter of water

- Optional: natural sweetener to taste

In a pot, boil the fenugreek seeds in water for 5-7 minutes. Add the ground cinnamon and let it steep for another 2 minutes. Strain the mixture and add honey or natural sweetener if desired.Fenugreek seeds are believed to improve insulin sensitivity, while cinnamon may help regulate blood sugar levels and boost metabolism.

8. Flaxseed and mint slimming infusion:

- 1 tablespoon ground flaxseed

- 1 handful of fresh mint leaves

- 1 liter of water

- Optional: A squeeze of fresh lime

juice

In a liter of water, combine the ground flaxseed and fresh mint leaves with water. Let it infuse inthe refrigerator for at least 2 hours. Add a squeeze of lime juice for extra flavor. Flaxseed is high in fiber and can aid in appetite control, while mint aids digestion and provides a refreshing taste.

9. Fennel Seed and Ginger Fat Burner:

- 1 teaspoon fennel seeds

- 1-inch piece of fresh ginger, grated or thinly sliced

- 1 litre of water

- Optional: A few drops of stevia extract or natural sweetener to taste

In a pot, boil the fennel seeds and ginger in water for 5-7 minutes. Strain the mixture and let it cool. Add a few drops of stevia extract or natural sweetener if desired. Fennel seeds may help reduce cravings, while ginger aids digestion and boosts metabolism.

Remember that while these fat-burning drinks may offer potential benefits, they are not instant solutions for weight loss. For effective and sustainable weight management, combine these drinks with a balanced diet, regular exercise, and a healthy lifestyle.

Note

As always, consult with a healthcare professional before making significant changes to your diet, especially if you have any underlying health conditions.